PHARMACIST HUMOR

IRENE XANDERENA

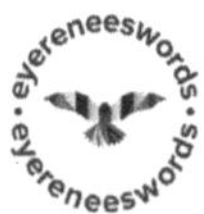

PHARMACIST HUMOR
Copyright © 2023, Irene Xanderena
All Rights Reserved.

No part of this publication may be reproduced, stored in a retrieval system, or transmitted in any form or by any means: Electronic, Mechanical, Photocopying, Recording, or otherwise, without prior written permission of the copyright owner or the publishers.

ISBN: 979-8-8690-1476-4

Published by
Eyereneeswords
Email: life@eyereneeswords.com
Website: www.eyereneeswords.com

CONTENT

ACKNOWLEDGMENT

I would like to express my gratitude to the pharmacists who have inspired me to write this humor book. Their dedication, hard work, and ability to handle challenging situations with grace and humor have been a true inspiration.

I also want to acknowledge the countless hours that pharmacists spend on their feet, tirelessly serving patients and ensuring their well-being. Without their commitment and expertise, our healthcare system would not function effectively. I would like to thank the pharmacists who have generously shared their humorous stories and anecdotes, allowing me to bring their experiences to life in this book.

Additionally, I want to acknowledge the importance of humor in our lives, especially during times of stress and uncertainty. By writing this humor book, I hope to bring smiles and laughter to both pharmacists and readers, reminding us all of the healing power of humor.

Finally, I want to thank my family, friends, and loved ones for their unwavering support and encouragement throughout this writing journey. Their belief in my project and their willingness to lend an ear during the brainstorming process have been invaluable.

Lastly, I want to express my gratitude to the readers who will embark on this humorous journey with me. It is my sincere desire that this book will provide a lighthearted escape and a shared moment of laughter, reminding us all to find joy in the everyday moments of life.

INTRODUCTION

I started writing the humor series in 2023 and after interviewing people of various professions, I gathered that Individuals tend to approach their lives and careers with great seriousness. So, I am injecting some much-needed laughter into everyone's life and career path. I have had the privilege of working with my sister, Anne Moji Williams, a pharmacist, and I understand the unique challenges that come with the job. I recognize how hard pharmacists work to keep us healthy.

Humor is a powerful tool for connection and understanding. With this humor book about pharmacists, I aim to shed light on the often-overlooked experiences of pharmacists while also providing a source of entertainment and levity. Through witty anecdotes and humorous observations, I hope to bridge the gap between pharmacists and the general public, offering a deeper appreciation for the important work pharmacists do. Furthermore, I hope to remind everyone of the resilience and good-natured humor that exists within the profession. I hope to bring a sense of joy and entertainment to readers everywhere.

A pharmacist is a healthcare professional who specializes in the preparation, dispensation, and monitoring of medications. They are responsible for ensuring the safe and effective use of medications by patients. Pharmacists have extensive knowledge of drug interactions, dosage guidelines, and potential side effects, making them essential members of the healthcare team.

With this book, I want to honor the countless pharmacists whose tireless work often goes unnoticed. It is my hope that through laughter and lightheartedness, I can help to create a greater appreciation for the world of pharmacy.

Pharmacists often face long hours, demanding patients, and the pressure to ensure the accuracy of medications, making their jobs incredibly stressful. By injecting humor into their experiences, I hope to provide them with a well-deserved break and a chance to laugh at the absurdities of their profession. Additionally, I aim to bring awareness to the unique challenges pharmacists face, as their work is often overshadowed by other healthcare professionals.

I expect to shed light on the behind-the-scenes world of pharmacy, revealing the humor that exists within it. Furthermore, I believe that humor has the power to connect people, and by sharing humorous jokes, I aspire to foster a sense of camaraderie among pharmacy professionals and create a space for shared experiences. Ultimately, my goal is to entertain and uplift both pharmacists and readers alike, while also highlighting the invaluable role that pharmacists play in our healthcare system.

UNIVERSAL PHARMACY SYMBOL

There are two recognized universal symbols for pharmacy. Picture this: a towering, majestic mortar and pestle, standing proudly as a beacon of hope and health. This iconic symbol features a large mortar, a vessel traditionally used for grinding and preparing medicines, accompanied by a pestle, the tool used to crush and mix ingredients.

Together, they form the timeless emblem that represents the world of pharmacy. Now, imagine this symbol adorned with a mischievous smile, a pair of friendly googly eyes, and perhaps even a tiny pharmacist's hat perched atop it. After all, why not add a touch of whimsy to an already iconic image? So, my friend, whether you spot this symbol on a sign, a storefront, or even on the side of a pill bottle, know that you've arrived at the gateway of healing, where the magic of pharmacy awaits.

The second symbol is the Rod of Asclepius, the snake pharmacy symbol! Picture this: a single snake, coiled around a staff with a winged top. This ancient symbol is associated with the Greek god Asclepius, who was revered as the god of healing and medicine. The Rod of Asclepius has become widely recognized as a symbol of the medical and healthcare professions. It is often used to represent pharmacies, hospitals, and other healthcare institutions. The snake is believed to symbolize rebirth and healing, while the staff represents authority and power.

It is important to note that sometimes the Rod of Asclepius is confused with the Caduceus, which features two snakes entwined around a staff with wings at the top. While the Caduceus is also a well-known symbol, it is more commonly associated with commerce and trade rather than medicine. So, when you spot the snake pharmacy symbol, know that it represents the noble art of healing and the dedication of those in the pharmacy profession to help others on their path toward wellness.

PREFACE

I am writing a humor book about pharmacists because I believe laughter, even in the pharmacy world, is the best prescription. Pharmacists often encounter unique situations and interactions that can be ripe for comedic storytelling. Additionally, humor can serve as a coping mechanism for the challenges pharmacists face, providing a lighthearted escape. Ultimately, my goal is to celebrate them and bring laughter to an often-underappreciated profession. Pharmacists play a crucial role in healthcare, yet their daily experiences are rarely highlighted in a comedic light. Through witty anecdotes and humorous observations, I want to shed light on the unique hilarious thoughts of pharmacists.

Having spent well over a decade working in the healthcare industry, I have witnessed the dedication, expertise, and occasional absurdity that comes with being a pharmacist. Moreover, humor can serve as a powerful coping mechanism for the challenges pharmacists face daily. The ability to find humor in the midst of stress and pressure can provide much-needed relief and foster a positive work environment. Let us celebrate the often unsung heroes behind the pharmacy counter. It is a testament to the professionalism, resilience, and good-natured humor that pharmacists bring to their work. Through laughter and lightheartedness, I want to bring joy, entertainment, and a newfound appreciation for the world of pharmacy to readers everywhere. So, my friend, hold onto your mortar and pestle, because we're about to embark on a laughter-filled journey as you read "Pharmacist Humor."

PHARMACIST
HUMOR

1

Why did the pharmacist become a magician?

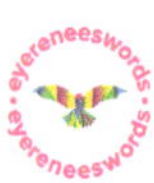

To turn pills into thoughts!

2

How does a pharmacist respond to stupid questions?

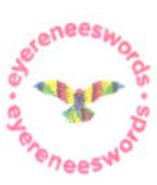

They hand out "I'm Sorry for Your Ignorance" pamphlets!

3

Why did the pharmacist become a comedian?

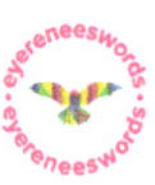

Because they had the perfect prescription for laughter!

4

How did the pharmacist know the patient was a math teacher?

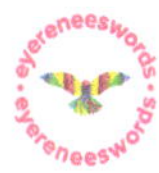

They had a prescription for square roots!

5

Why did the pharmacist study music theory?

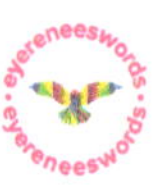

To understand the prescription of harmony!

6

How do pharmacists make decisions?

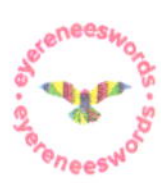

They always weigh the pros and prescriptions!

7

What did the pharmacist say to the patient who couldn't pronounce their medication?

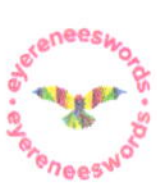

"Don't worry, it's just a tongue twister!"

8

Why did the pharmacist bring a ladder to work?

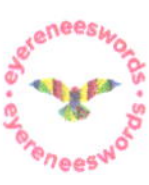

To reach the price of the high prescriptions.

9

Why did the pharmacist become a pharmacist?

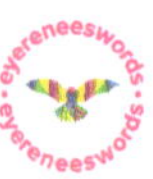

They couldn't find a job dispensing soda!

10

What do you call
a pharmacist who
works at night?

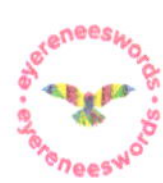

A nocturnal druggist!

11

Why do pharmacists always
win at poker?

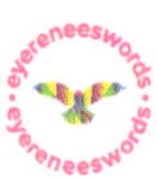

Because they know when
to hold 'em and when
to fold 'em!

12

What do you call a pharmacist who is also a rapper?

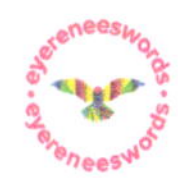

A pill-er!

13

Why did the pharmacist go broke?

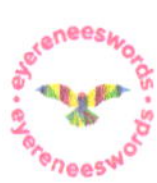

They lost their common cents!

14

What do you call a pharmacist who accidentally dispenses too many painkillers?

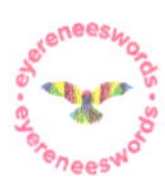

An aspirin' entrepreneur!

15

Why do pharmacists become stand-up comedians?

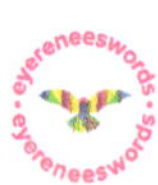

Because they have a knack for dispensing punchlines!

16

Why did the pharmacist
get promoted?

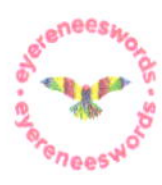

Because they are good at
dispensing advice!

17

Why do pharmacists become gardeners?

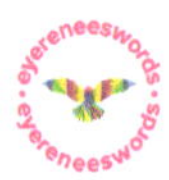

Because they love working with herb-al remedies!

18

Why did the pharmacist's computer go to the doctor?

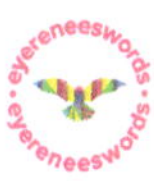

It had a virus and needed a prescription!

19

What did the pharmacist say to the annoying customer?

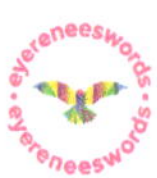

"Sir, patience is not an over-the-counter medication."

20

Why did the pharmacist become an archaeologist?

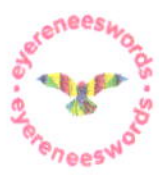

Because they loved digging up ancient remedies!

21

What do you call a pharmacist who loves to dance?

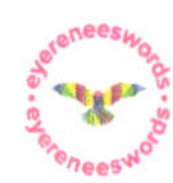

A Pillarina!

22

Why did the pharmacist get a pet parrot?

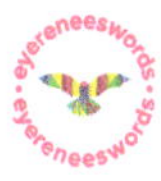

As a reminder to always "Rx-spect the customer's needs!"

23

How do pharmacists handle difficult customers?

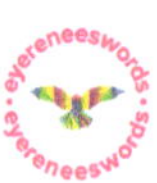

They always keep a steady dose of professionalism!

24

Why did the pharmacist become a gardener?

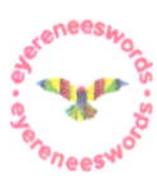

To learn the art of cultivating drug plants!

25

What do you call a pharmacist who knows how to mix the perfect cocktail?

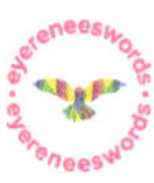

A "pharma-cistern"

26

What did the pharmacist say to the customer who couldn't remember their prescription?

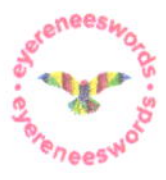

"It's time to refill your memory!

27

What do you call a
pharmacist who loves to fish?

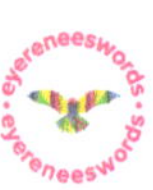

A "pharma-cologist"!

28

Why did the pharmacist become an artist?

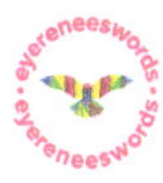

He loved the idea of creating "prescription masterpieces"!

29

How do pharmacists solve problems?

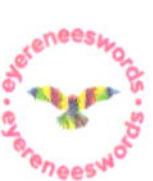

With a "prescription for success"!

30

What do you call
a pharmacist who
loves puzzles?

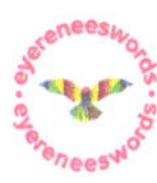

A "riddle-a-cist!

31

Why did the pharmacist
become a magician?

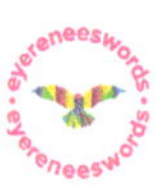

To make medications appear,
and then disappear.

32

What did the pharmacist say to the customer who asked for a discount?

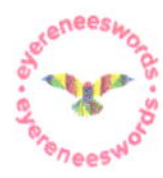

"I'll have to charge you a dis-count-sultation fee!"

33

How do you spot
a pharmacist at a
vacation resort?

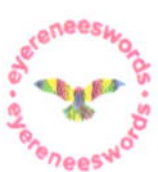

You hear them having "pillow
talk" with their medications–
discussing drug interactions,
side effects, and dosages.

34

A Pharmacist is like a modern-day wizard!

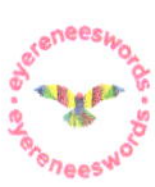

They have the ability to transform a doctor's prescription into a tangible and effective medication. They are very powerful!

35

Pharmacists are spelling bee champions!

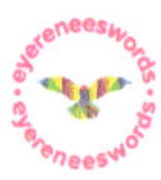

They will spell the generic and brand name of your medication and pronounce it without tongue-twisting.

36

Step back, accountants!
Pharmacists are the counting
pros! They never miss a
pill count!

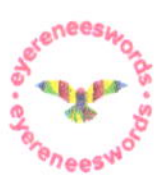

37

Pharmacists are expert mixologists, but instead of cocktails, they're making personalized medications!

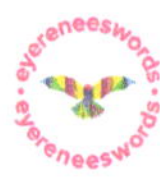

38

Why did the pharmacist become a comedian?

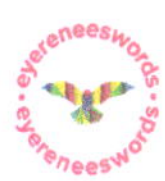

Because they have the "pills" to make everyone laugh!

39

Why did the pharmacist refuse to play cards?

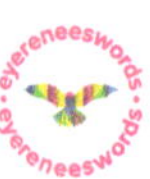

He was too afraid of "drug" interactions!

40

What did the pharmacist say to the impatient customer?

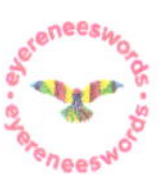

"Don't worry, I have a "prescription" for your impatience!"

41

Why did the pretty pharmacist always have a great sense of humor?

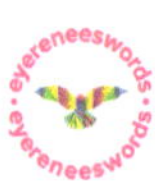

She gave herself a "dose" of laughter with every prescription!

42

How did the pharmacist know the patient was a math teacher?

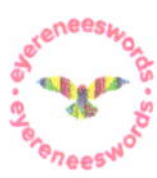

He always came in with a "counting problem"!

43

Pharmacists are like superheroes, but instead of capes, they wear lab coats and carry pill bottles!

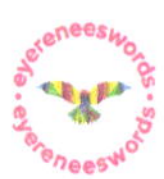

44

You know you're a pharmacist in the making when you can spell medication names better than you can spell your own name!

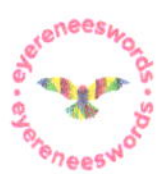

45

Pharmacists deal with so many medications that they probably dream in prescription codes!

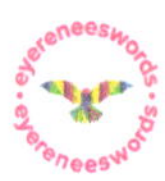

46

If you can make a pharmacist laugh, you can't be human!

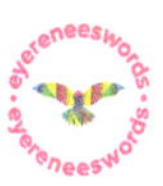

47

Pharmacists know that the real magic happens behind the counter, and not in the wizarding world of Harry Potter!

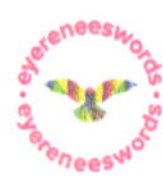

48

Pharmacists are the true masters of multitasking. You have 10 different prescriptions? They got you!

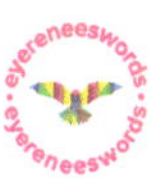

49

Pharmacists will read every drug interaction and stop your doctor's prescription from ending you.

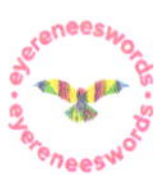

50

What do you call a group of pharmacists on a road trip?

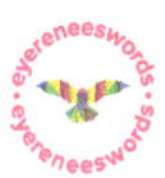

A "prescription" for adventure!

51

How do pharmacists like their coffee?

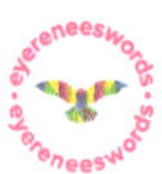

Strong, coated with a "shot" of placebo and a side effect of humor!

52

How do pharmacists like to relax?

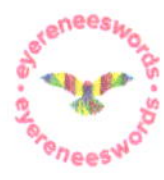

By taking a "pill-ow" and getting a good night's sleep!

53

What did the pharmacist say to the patient who couldn't stop cracking bad jokes?

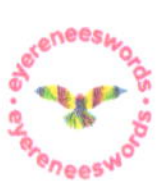

"You need a new prescription!

54

Do you know what pharmacists think of some prescription interactions after drinking their third cup of coffee?

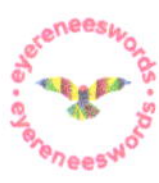

Even the strongest coffee can't fix stupid prescriptions!"

55

What did the comedian say
to the crowd?

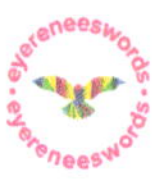

I'm like a pharmacist, but
with a sense of humor. I
dispense laughter instead
of pills!"

56

Pharmacy tip: Laughter is the best medicine, so take a dose of my jokes and call me in the morning!"

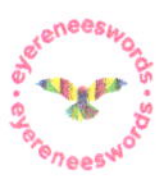

57

"I'm the pharmacist who can turn your frown upside down, even if your prescription label says 'serious side effects.'"

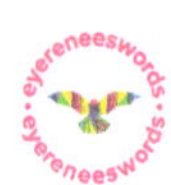

58

They say laughter
is contagious, but so
are my medication
recommendations!

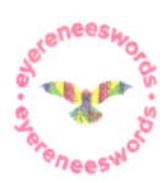

59

Pharmacists: the only professionals who can count pills without taking their shoes off!"

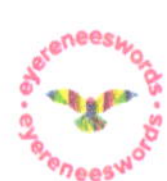

60

We may be quiet, but
our knowledge of
medication is louder than a
marching band!"

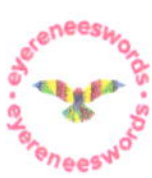

61

We may not have a magic wand, but we can make your medication disappear without a trace!"

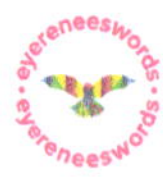

62

Pharmacists: the unofficial therapists of the pharmacy world, listening to people's prescription problems and giving out free smiles!"

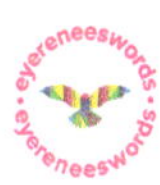

63

Pharmacists: the masters of multitasking, juggling prescriptions, and pretending to understand doctor's handwriting!"

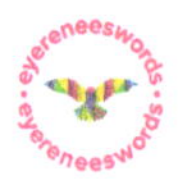

64

If pharmacists had their way, they would prescribe a bottle of "anti-social" pills to talkative customers.

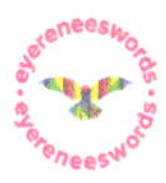

65

Watch the pharmacist put on a fake smile and say, "How can I help?" and pretend like they care.

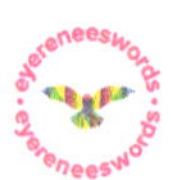

66

Some pharmacists have a special talent for making customers disappear with just a glare.

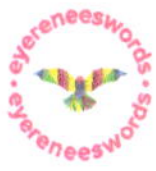

67

What did the pharmacist prescribe for a husband who has a talkative wife?

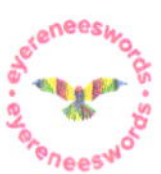

He suggested a medication that caused temporary hearing loss.

68

When a customer would not stop talking, the pharmacist offered them a free subscription to a "No Social Interaction" magazine.

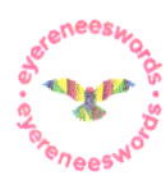

69

When people come to the pharmacist to argue about their prescription, the pharmacist responds with a blank stare and a shrug.

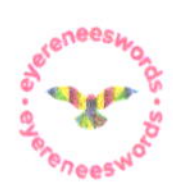

70

Whenever a customer complained about the prescription prices, the pharmacist would respond with "Well, if you don't like it, I can prescribe you a sense of humor."

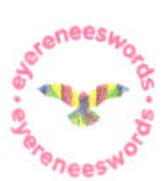

71

Whenever a talkative customer enters the store, the pharmacist puts on noise-canceling headphones and starts miming instead of speaking.

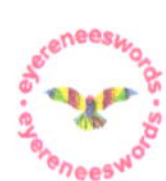

72

Instead of offering a loyalty program, the pharmacist offers a "Silent Shopper" discount for those who shop without saying a word.

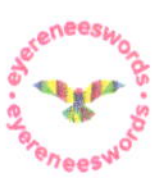

73

Instead of giving out free samples, the pharmacist gives out free earplugs to customers, just in case they feel the urge to start a conversation.

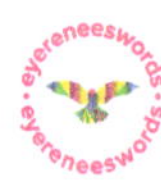

74

How do you make a
pharmacist laugh?

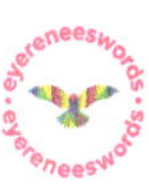

Just give them a placebo and
tell them it's a brand-new
wonder drug!

75

How do pharmacists like their martini?

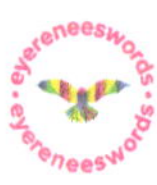

Just like their prescriptions– strong and well-dosed!

76

Why did the pharmacist become a hermit?

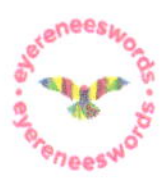

They preferred the company of pill bottles over people!

77

What did the pharmacist say when asked why they don't talk to patients?

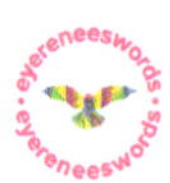

Well, I deal with prescriptions, not personalities!"

78

What's a pharmacist's motto?

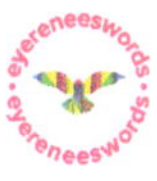

"Prescriptions, not people.

79

Why did the pharmacist become a pharmacist?

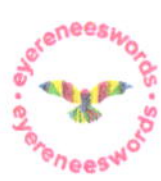

Because they wanted to be surrounded by pill bottles instead of people with problems!

80

How does a pharmacist greet customers?

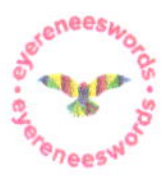

With a fake smile and a hidden eye roll!

81

How does a pharmacist handle chatty customers?

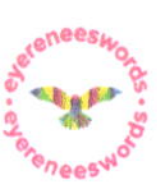

They give them an "over-the-counter" recommendation for a good therapist!

82

How does a pharmacist react to a customer's complaints?

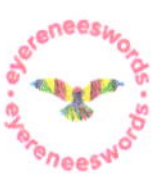

They just smile while thinking: "Hey, at least I'm not the one with the prescription for attitude adjustment!"

83

What's a pharmacist's secret talent?

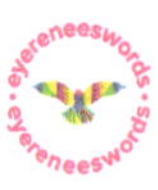

The ability to calculate the exact amount of time it takes for a customer to annoy them!

84

What's a pharmacist's favorite game?

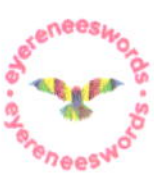

"Counting Pills" – the more they count, the less they have to interact with customers!

85

How does a pharmacist react to a customer's complaints?

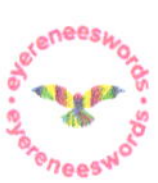

They just nod politely and think, "If only there was a pill to cure entitled behavior!"

86

How does a pharmacist handle talkative customers?

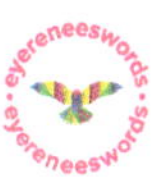

They give them a prescription for a "Mute Button" to take before each conversation!

87

What did the pharmacist say to the talkative customer's wife?

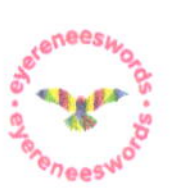

Before you go home, you will probably need a prescription for patience.

88

What's a pharmacist's
favorite song?

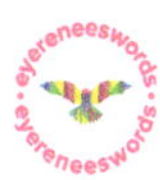

"Don't Stand So Close to Me"
by The Police.

89

What's a pharmacist's idea of a nightmare?

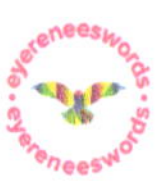

Being trapped in a crowded room full of customers who never stop talking.

90

Why did the pharmacist start wearing a "Do Not Disturb" sign around their neck?

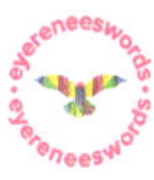

To signal to customers that they're not interested in engaging in conversation.

91

How does a pharmacist handle a chatty customer?

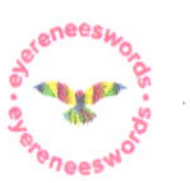

They start speaking in medical jargon until the customer gets confused and leaves.

92

How does a pharmacist handle a demanding customer?

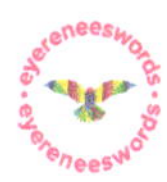

They give them a prescription for a reality check.

93

What's a pharmacist's favorite saying to rude customers?

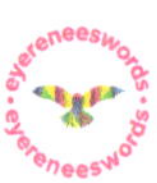

I'm sorry, we don't have a magic pill to fix your attitude."

94

Why did the pharmacist start practicing yoga?

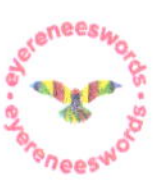

To find their inner calm before dealing with infuriating customers.

95

What's a pharmacist's secret weapon?

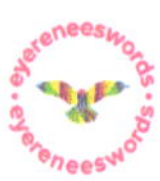

The ability to deliver a sarcastic response without getting caught!

10 HEALTH TIPS FROM PHARMACISTS

1. **Take medications as prescribed:** Pharmacists emphasize the importance of following medication instructions to ensure optimal effectiveness and minimize potential side effects.

2. **Consult a pharmacist for over-the-counter (OTC) medication advice:** Pharmacists possess extensive knowledge about various OTC medications and can provide guidance on selecting the right product for your specific needs.

3. **Keep an updated medication list:** Maintaining an accurate list of all medications, including prescription, OTC, and supplements, helps pharmacists identify potential drug interactions and ensure your safety.

4. **Practice proper medication storage:** Pharmacists recommend storing medications in a cool, dry place, away from direct sunlight and out of reach of children and pets, to maintain their potency and prevent accidental ingestion.

5. **Stay current with vaccinations:** Pharmacists can provide information and administer immunizations, helping you stay protected against preventable diseases.

6. **Seek pharmacist advice for managing side effects:** If you experience adverse effects from medications, consulting a pharmacist can offer guidance on managing symptoms or exploring alternative options.

7. **Dispose of medications properly:** Pharmacists can guide you on safe medication disposal methods to prevent environmental contamination and accidental ingestion.

8. **Ask about medication adherence aids:** Pharmacists can recommend tools such as pill organizers or smartphone apps to help you stay organized and remember to take medications as prescribed.

9. **Be proactive in medication reviews:** Regularly consulting with a pharmacist for medication reviews can help identify any potential issues, such as duplicate therapies or drug interactions, ensuring optimal medication management.

10. **Take advantage of pharmacist counseling services:** Pharmacists are not only medication experts but also valuable sources of health information. Utilize their counseling services to address any concerns, ask questions, or seek advice on various health-related topics.

10 REASONS WE NEED A PHARMACIST

1. **Medication expertise:** Pharmacists possess in-depth knowledge of medications, their uses, side effects, and interactions, ensuring safe and effective treatment.

2. **Patient counseling:** Pharmacists educate patients about their medications, including proper usage, potential risks, and strategies for adherence, promoting optimal health outcomes.

3. **Drug safety:** Pharmacists play a crucial role in preventing medication errors, ensuring accurate dosing, and identifying potential drug interactions or allergies.

4. **Prescription verification:** Pharmacists carefully review prescriptions to ensure accuracy, appropriateness, and compatibility

with a patient's medical history, preventing potential harm.

5. **Medication management:** Pharmacists help patients manage complex medication regimens, improving adherence and minimizing the risk of missed doses or drug-related complications.

6. **Chronic disease management:** Pharmacists contribute to the management of chronic conditions by providing specialized medication counseling and monitoring, helping patients achieve better control of their health.

7. **Immunization services:** Pharmacists are trained to administer vaccines, increasing access to immunizations and promoting public health initiatives.

8. **Drug information resource:** Pharmacists are valuable sources of drug information for healthcare professionals, assisting in decision-

making, and providing evidence-based recommendations.

9. **Drug therapy optimization:** Pharmacists collaborate with healthcare teams to optimize drug therapy, ensuring the most effective and cost-efficient treatments are prescribed.

10. **Community health promotion:** Pharmacists actively engage in health promotion campaigns, providing education on topics such as smoking cessation, contraception, and preventative measures, contributing to overall community well-being.